REVERSING CHRONIC KIDNEY DISEASE

HOW TO MAINTAIN KIDNEY HEALTH AND PREVENT UNDERGOING DIALYSIS

BY

LAURA WARREN, M.D

Table of Contents

Introduction

No matter what the reason, constant kidney sickness is described by the presence of kidney harm or diminished kidney capability for no less than 90 days. As per the Kidney Illness further developing world-wide results rules, a diminished assessed glomerular filtration rate and no less than one marker of kidney harm (albuminuria, underlying irregularities, irregularities in pee residue, electrolyte anomalies, and a past filled with kidney transplantation) for something like three months are expected for finding.

However, glomerulonephritis is another possibility. In order to determine the cause, the initial workup should include a comprehensive medical history, physical examination, blood pressure history, dietary history, weight measurements, serum electrolytes, fasting lipids, glycated hemoglobin (HbA1c), and urine albumin/creatinine ratio. Stage 1-5, which is determined by GFR and albuminuria level, is characterized by obesity, smoking, high blood pressure, and other risk factors.

According to clinical guidelines, kidney failure progresses when a patients GFR falls below 15 mL/min/1.73 m2, when they require dialysis, or when they need a transplant. End-stage renal sickness doesnt necessarily in every case go with kidney disappointment. The definition of ESRD, which is used by health insurance to describe patients who are on dialysis or transplantation, does not include kidney failure patients who are not on dialysis or transplantation.

Chapter 1

The Problem of Kidney Disease

The gradual loss of kidney function is a hallmark of chronic kidney disease, which is also known as chronic kidney failure. Your kidneys purify your blood to get rid of wastes and excess fluids, which are then thrown out in your urine. With advanced chronic kidney disease, your body can build up dangerous amounts of fluid, electrolytes, and waste. There may not be many warning signs or symptoms in the early stages of chronic kidney disease. You might not be aware that you have kidney disease until it is too late. Treatment for chronic kidney disease typically aims to control the underlying cause to stop kidney damage from getting worse.

However, controlling the cause may not be sufficient to prevent kidney damage from worsening. Dialysis or a kidney transplant is not necessary for end-stage kidney failure, which is lethal in chronic kidney disease. Chronic kidney disease manifests over time if damage to the kidneys progresses slowly. A decline in kidney function can lead to an accumulation of fluid, body waste, or electrolyte imbalances. Depending on the severity, kidney function loss can result in the following:

At the point when liquid develops in the lungs or around the hearts covering, it can cause windedness and chest torment, the two of which are indications of kidney sickness. Nausea, vomiting, a lack of appetite, fatigue, and weakness are additional symptoms.

Urinary incontinence can also be brought on by sleep issues. Kidney disease can also cause muscle cramps and dry, itchy skin. This shows that they may likewise be welcomed on by different infections. Because your kidneys are able to make up for lost function, you may not experience symptoms until damage has become irreversible.

When To See A Doctor

Kidney disease symptoms should prompt a visit to the doctor. Early detection of kidney disease can stop it from progressing to kidney failure. Assuming you have an ailment that builds your gamble of kidney illness, your PCP might lead pee and blood tests during your exam to screen your circulatory strain and kidney capability.

At the point when an illness or condition influences kidney capability and makes harm deteriorate more than a while or years, this is called persistent kidney sickness. The following diseases and conditions can result in chronic kidney disease: Diabetes, high blood pressure, and either type 1 or type 2 diabetes Glomerulonephritis, an inflammation of the kidneys filtering units (glomeruli) Interstitial nephritis, an inflammation of the kidneys tubules and surrounding structures.

Polycystic kidney disease or other inherited kidney diseases Prolonged urinary tract obstruction caused by conditions like an enlarged prostate, kidney stones, and some cancers Vesicoureteral reflux, a

condition that causes urine to a few potential issues
include:

- Damage to your central nervous system,
  which can cause difficulty concentrating,
  personality changes, or seizures.
- Damage to your immune system, which
  makes you more susceptible to infection.
- Pericarditis, an inflammation of the
  saclike membrane that envelops your
  heart (pericardium).
- Complications during pregnancy that
  carry risks for the mother and the
  developing fetus Irreversible damage.
- Prescription medications should be taken
  as directed. Follow the instructions on the
  package when taking nonprescription
  painkillers like acetaminophen (Tylenol)
  and ibuprofen (Advil, Motrin IB, and
  others) for headaches.
- If you take too many painkillers for a long
  time, it could hurt your kidneys.

Maintain A Healthy Weight

Engage in regular physical activity to keep your weight in a healthy range. If you need to lose weight, talk to your doctor about healthy options.

Dont Smoke

Smoking can cause damage to your kidneys or worsen existing damage. In the event that you smoke, converse with your PCP about ways of stopping. Counseling, medication, and support groups can all assist you in quitting.

Utilize The Assistance Of Your Physician To Manage Your Medical Conditions

 Manage any conditions or diseases that put you at risk for kidney disease with your doctors help. Your doctor can order tests to look for signs of kidney damage.

What Is a kidney Failure

When one or both of your kidneys stop working normally on their own, this condition is known as renal failure. In some instances, kidney failure can be brief and swift (acute). Sometimes its a condition that gets worse over time and lasts a long time.

When one or both of your kidneys cease to function normally, you have kidney failure. The causes include acute kidney injuries, diabetes, and high blood pressure. The treatments are dialysis or a kidney transplant. The most severe stage of kidney disease is kidney failure. Without treatment, it is fatal. Without treatment, kidney failure patients may survive for a few days or weeks.

How Does The kidneys Function?

Your kidneys are bean-molded organs about the size of your clench hand. They are positioned toward your back, under your ribcage. The vast majority have two working kidneys, however you can live well with just a single kidney for however long its working accurately.

The kidneys perform multiple tasks. Helping your body get rid of toxins is one of the most important jobs. Your kidneys are responsible for filtering your blood and exchanging waste products with urine. Your body builds up waste products when your kidney doesn't work right. Assuming this occurs, youll feel wiped out and in the long run bite the dust without treatment. With the right treatment, kidney failure is manageable for many people.

When Kidney Failure Begins, What Happens?

Depending on your estimated glomerular filtration rate (eGFR), there are stages of kidney disease. A calculation of how well your kidneys filter substances is your eGFR. An average eGFR is close to 100. When the eGFR falls to zero, there is no kidney function left. Any kidney disease has stages, which include:

Stage I: You have a GFR that is above 90 but below 100. Your kidneys are only slightly damaged at this point, but they still work normally.

Stage 2: Your GFR might be essentially as low as 60 or as high as 89. Your kidneys are damaged more than they were in stage I, but they still work well.

Stage 3: Your GFR can be anywhere from 30 to 59. You might have gentle or serious loss of kidney capability.

Stage 4: Your GFR can be anywhere from 15 to 29. Your kidney function has seriously deteriorated.

Stage 5: Your GFR is below 15 and your kidneys are either close to or completely failing.

Symptoms And Causes

Many people with kidney disease experience few or
no symptoms at first. Even if you feel fine, chronic
kidney disease can still cause damage, and kidney
failure symptoms vary from person to person. One
or more of the following symptoms may occur if
your kidneys arent working properly:

- Extreme exhaustion (fatigue)
- Diabetes
- Indigestion and vomiting
- Confusion or difficulty focusing
- Edema, or swelling, especially around your hands, ankles, or face.
- More frequently peeing.
- Muscle spasms, or cramps
- Skin that is dry or achy
- A lack of appetite or metallic food may taste.
- Kidney disease in the family.
- A previous kidney damage.
- You take NSAIDs frequently.

Hyperglycemia, or high blood sugar levels, can result from uncontrolled diabetes. The kidneys and other organs can be harmed by consistently high glucose levels. Hypertension implies blood voyages powerfully through your bodys veins. If you dont get treatment, the extra force could cause tissue damage to your kidneys over time.

In most cases, kidney failure does not occur quickly. Other factors that could result in kidney failure are:

PKD, or polycystic kidney disease PKD is a condition you acquire from one of your folks (acquired condition) that causes liquid filled sacs (blisters) to develop inside your kidneys.

Diseases Of The Glomerule

Kidney function is affected by glomerular diseases lupus. In addition to organ damage, joint pain, fever, and skin rashes, lupus is an autoimmune disease. A sudden occurrence can also precipitate kidney failure quickly. When your kidneys suddenly stop working, this is called acute kidney failure or acute kidney injury. Within a matter of hours or days, acute kidney failure may occur. It is frequently brief.

The following are typical causes of acute kidney failure:

- Kidney disease caused by an immune system reaction.
- A few medications.
- Severe lack of water.
- Obstruction of the urinary tract.
- Systemic diseases that go untreated, like liver or heart disease.

Does Kidney Failure Spread?

No, kidney disappointment isnt infectious.
Additionally, you cannot spread conditions that
cause to another individual.

How Is Kidney Disappointment Analyzed?

To evaluate your kidneys and diagnose kidney
failure, a healthcare provider may use a variety of
kidney function tests. Common tests that the doctor
may order if they think you are at risk for kidney
failure include:

A Blood Test

The efficiency with which your kidneys remove
waste from your blood is determined by blood tests.
A provider will take a small amount of blood from a
vein in your arm with a thin needle. At a laboratory,
technicians will then examine your blood sample.

Urinalysis Test

Specific substances in your urine, like protein or blood, are measured in urine tests. At a doctors office or a hospital, you will urinate in a special container. In a laboratory, technicians will then examine your urine sample.

Tests of Images

A doctor can look at your kidneys and the areas around them with imaging tests to find problems or obstructions. Ultrasound of the kidney, a CT urogram, and an MRI are all common types of imaging tests.

The treatment for kidney failure depends on the nature and severity of the problem.
Therapy for a constant ailment can dial back the movement of kidney illness. In the event that your kidneys gradually stop working, your doctor or nurse might use a few different approaches to monitor your health and keep your kidneys working as long as possible. Some of these methods include:

- ☐ Periodic blood tests.
- ☐ Controls of blood pressure.

☐   Medication.

Treatment is needed to keep you alive if you have kidney failure. There are two ways to treat kidney failure.
Dialysis enables the body to filter blood while Hemodialysis which is a machine regularly cleans your blood. The vast majority get hemodialysis three to four days per week at a clinic or dialysis facility. peritoneal dialysis.

A catheter is inserted into your abdominal lining during peritoneal dialysis, and a bag containing the dialysis solution is attached to it. The arrangement streams from the sack into your stomach lining, retains side-effects and additional liquids and channels once more into the pack. Now and then individuals can get peritoneal dialysis at home.

During a kidney transplant, a surgeon inserts a healthy kidney into your body to replace the damaged one. A living donor or a deceased donor can provide the healthy kidney, also known as the donor organ. With just one healthy kidney, you can live happily. Indeed, you can recuperate from kidney disappointment with appropriate treatment. You might require treatment until the end of your life.

How Long Can Kidney Failure Keep You Alive?

Kidney breakdown is destructive without dialysis or a kidney transplant. May survive without treatment for a few days or weeks.
The typical dialysis patient lives for five to ten years. On dialysis, some people can live for up to 30 years.
The average life expectancy of a kidney transplant recipient from a living donor is 12 to 20 years. If you receive a kidney from a deceased donor, you can expect to live anywhere from eight to twelve years.

What Meds Are Utilized To Treat Kidney Disappointment?

One or more of the following medications may be prescribed to you by your healthcare provider depending on the cause of your kidney disease:

1.Angiotensin II receptor blocker (ARB) or inhibitor of the angiotensin-converting enzyme (ACE)

Your blood pressure will fall as a result of these medications.
Diuretics. These aid in the removal of extra fluid from the body.

2. Statins

Reduce your cholesterol levels with these substances that stimulate erythropoietin. If you have anemia, these aid in the production of red blood cells.
Vitamin D and calcitriol. These assist in halting bone loss.

3. Binders with phosphate

These assist in eliminating extra phosphorus from your blood.

Prevention

Even though kidney failure is irreversible, you can help keep your kidneys working. Your kidneys ability to function may decline more slowly if you maintain healthy routines and habits. If you have kidney failure, you should do the following:

Keep an eye on your kidney health.
If you have diabetes, keep your blood sugar levels within normal range.
Maintain a normal level of blood pressure.
Stay away from tobacco products.
Stay away from food sources high in protein and sodium.
Attend each and every appointment that your healthcare provider has scheduled for you.

However, kidney failure cannot be treated.
However, you may still live a long life with minimal

impact on your quality of life if you receive the appropriate diagnosis and treatment.

Chapter 2

Natural methods for treating and reversing chronic kidney disease

Preventing Chronic Kidney Disease If you have diabetes, high blood pressure, heart disease, or a family history of kidney failure, you are more likely to develop kidney disease.

What can I do to ensure the good health of my kidneys?

Diabetes and high blood pressure, two conditions that can damage the kidneys, can be avoided or controlled to protect them. Your kidneys, as well as the rest of your body, may benefit from following the steps listed below.
You might want to inquire about your kidney health at your next medical appointment.

Getting tested may be the only way to determine whether your kidneys are in good health because early kidney disease may not have any symptoms.

The frequency of your tests will be determined with your providers assistance.

If you develop a urinary tract infection (UTI), which if left untreated can harm your kidneys, see a provider right away.

Choose foods that are good for your heart and body as a whole when it comes to eating: whole grains, fresh fruits, vegetables, either fresh or frozen, and dairy products with low or no fat.

Reduce your intake of salt and added sugars and eat healthy meals.

Try to consume no more than 2,300 milligrams of sodium per day.

 Attempt to have under 10% of your everyday calories come from added sugars. Select foods that are good for your health.

Tips For Choosing Healthy Foods

- ☐ Replace salt with a mix of spices

- For your pizza, add peppers, spinach, and broccoli as veggie toppings.

- Have a go at baking or searing meat, chicken, and fish as opposed to broiling.

- Serve dishes without gravy or fats added.

- Try to select foods that contain very little or no added sugar.

- Start with whole milk and work your way down to 2% milk until you can drink and cook with fat-free (skim) or low-fat milk and products.

- Eat food varieties produced using entire grains like entire wheat, earthy colored rice, oats, and entire grain corn consistently.

- Sandwiches and toast should be made with whole-grain bread.

- White rice can be substituted for brown rice in both home-cooked meals and dining out.

Read The Food Labels

Choose foods that are low in cholesterol, trans fats, saturated fat, sodium, salt, and added sugars. At snack time, slow down. A slice of cake takes less time to eat than a bag of low-fat popcorn. Instead of drinking orange juice, peel an orange and eat it.

Try Writing Down Everything You Eat For A Week

You might be able to see when you tend to eat too much or eat foods with a lot of calories or fat. The DASH eating plan from the NIH may help you lower your blood pressure, according to research.

Find And Work With A Dietitian
External link to create a meal plan that meets your needs if you have diabetes, high blood pressure, or heart disease.

Include Physical Activity In Your Daily Routine By Exercising For At Least 30 Minutes On Most Days: Ask your doctor about the kinds and amounts Of physical activity that are right for you if you are not currently active. These advice to get you moving will help you add more activity to your life.

Aim For A Healthy Weight: The online NIH Body Weight Planner can assist you in customizing your calorie and exercise plans to reach and maintain a healthy weight. In the event that you are

overweight or have stoutness, work with your medical care supplier or dietitian to make a sensible weight reduction plan. View additional resources for weight management and physical activity to help you stay motivated.

Get Enough Sleep

Each night, aim for 7 to 8 hours. Take steps to improve your sleeping habits if you have trouble falling asleep NIH external link.

Stop Using Tobacco

If you smoke or use other forms of tobacco. So you dont have to do it on your own, ask for help.

Limit Alcohol Consumption

NIH external link Drinking excessive amounts of alcohol can raise blood pressure and add calories, which can cause weight gain. On the off chance that you drink liquor Outside interface, restrict yourself to one beverage each day assuming you are a lady and two beverages each day assuming that you are a man. One beverage is: 12 ounces of beer, 5 ounces of wine, 1.5 ounces of liquor, and stress-relieving activities.

Explore Stress-Relieving Activities, Learn How To Manage Stress, Relax, And Deal With Problems Can Improve Emotional And Physical Health

Mind-body practices like meditation, yoga, and tai chi, as well as physical activity like running or swimming, can help alleviate stress.

Control Hypertension, Diabetes, And Heart Disease

 The best way to protect your kidneys from damage if you have diabetes, high blood pressure, or heart disease is to keep your blood glucose levels close to your goal. Monitoring your blood glucose, or blood sugar level, is an important part of managing your diabetes. Its possible that your medical team will require you to test your blood glucose at least once per day.

Keep your blood pressure close to your target The target blood pressure for most diabetics is 140/90 mm Hg. Find out more about the NIH external link for high blood pressure.

Accept every one of your meds as recommended: Converse with your medical care supplier about specific circulatory strain drugs, called Pro inhibitors and ARBs, which might safeguard your kidneys. These medications have the suffix -pril or -sartan in their names.

Avoid using over-the-counter painkillers on a daily basis. Your kidneys may become damaged if you take nonsteroidal anti-inflammatory drugs

(NSAIDs) on a regular basis, such as ibuprofen (NIH external link) and naproxen (NIH external link). Find out about over-the-counter drugs and your kidneys.

Keep your cholesterol levels within the recommended range to help prevent heart attacks and strokes. There are two kinds of cholesterol in your blood: Both LDL and HDL Your blood vessels can become clogged with LDL, or "bad" cholesterol, which can lead to a heart attack or stroke. HDL, or "good" cholesterol, aids in the elimination of "bad" cholesterol from blood vessels. Triglycerides, a different type of blood fat, can also be measured by a cholesterol test.

During your next medical appointment, ask your healthcare provider the following important questions about your kidney health. The sooner you are diagnosed with kidney disease, the sooner you can receive treatment to aid in kidney protection.

Questions you should ask your doctor:
- What is my glomerular filtration rate (GFR)?
- What is the result of my albuminuria?
- My blood pressure is what?

- [ ] For diabetics, what is my blood glucose level?
- [ ] How frequently should I have my kidneys examined?
- [ ] What can I do to ensure the health of my kidneys?
- [ ] Do I need to take other medications?
- [ ] Should I increase my physical activity?
- [ ] What kind of exercise can I do?
- [ ] What can I consume?
- [ ] Is my weight healthy?
- [ ] Do I have to chat with a dietitian to find support with dinner arranging?
- [ ] For my kidneys, should I take ARBs or ACE inhibitors?
- [ ] What occurs assuming I have kidney sickness?

Chapter 3

How diet can help improve kidney function

A kidney-friendly diet should focus on fruits, vegetables, whole grains, low-fat dairy, and lean meats (such as seafood, poultry, eggs, legumes, nuts, seeds, and soy products) instead of sodium, cholesterol, and fat.

The majority of people with advanced kidney disease should eat a diet that is good for the kidneys and helps reduce blood waste. A renal diet is a common name for this diet. Limit sodium intake to no more than 2,000 milligrams per day to aid in improving kidney function and preventing further damage.

Watching what you eat and drink is important if you have chronic kidney disease. This is because your kidneys are unable to properly remove fluid and waste from your body. A diet that is good for your kidneys can help you live a longer life.

What Kind of Diet Is Kidney-Friendly?

The kidneys are responsible for removing waste and excess fluid from the body through urination. Also, they check your bodys minerals, like potassium and salt, are balanced. Your bodys liquids are balanced. You make chemicals that affect how different organs work. A kidney-accommodating eating routine is an approach to eating that shields your kidneys from additional harm.

To prevent the accumulation of other minerals and fluids, such as electrolytes, in your body, you will need to restrict some foods and beverages. At the same time, youll need to make sure you get enough vitamins, minerals, protein, and calories.
Its possible that there arent any restrictions on what you can eat when youre in the early stages of However, as the disease progresses, you will need to exercise greater caution regarding the foods you consume.

You might work with a dietitian to select foods that are gentle on your kidneys, according to your doctor. They might suggest:

Reduce sodium intake This mineral is naturally
present in many foods. Table salt contains the most
of it. Your blood pressure is affected by sodium.
Additionally, it aids in maintaining your bodys
water balance. The kidneys in good health control
sodium levels.

 However, if you have, your body accumulates
fluids and additional sodium. This can cause various
issues, as enlarged lower legs, hypertension,
windedness, and liquid development around your
heart and lungs. In your daily diet, you should aim
for less than 2 grams of sodium.
Take these easy steps to reduce sodium intake:

High-sodium seasonings like garlic salt, soy sauce,
and table salt should be avoided.
Cook at home because most fast food contains a lot
of sodium.
Attempt new flavors and spices instead of salt.
If at all possible, stay away from packaged foods.
They typically have a lot of sodium.
When you shop, read the labels and choose foods
with low sodium.
Before serving, rinse canned vegetables, beans,
meats, and fish with water.

Limit calcium and phosphorus because your bones
need these minerals to be healthy and strong.
 The excess phosphorus that you dont need is taken
out of your body by healthy kidneys.

 However, assuming that your phosphorus levels can
get excessively high. You run the risk of heart
disease as a result. Additionally, your calcium levels
start to decrease. Your body extracts it from your
bones to make up for it. They might become weaker
and easier to break as a result.

Your doctor may suggest that you consume no more
than 1,000 milligrams (mg) of phosphorus mineral
each day if you have late-stage This can be done by:
Choosing foods with low phosphorus levels (look
for "PHOS" on the label), eating more fresh fruits
and vegetables, eating corn and rice cereal, drinking
light-colored soda, limiting dairy and processed
foods, and cutting back on meat, poultry, and fish.

Calcium-rich foods also tend to be high in
phosphorus. You might be told by the doctor to cut
back on calcium-rich foods. The following dairy
products have a lower phosphorus content:
Brie, Swiss, regular, low-fat cream cheese, or sour
cream Sherbet. Your doctor may also advise you to

stop taking calcium supplements purchased over the counter and prescribe a phosphorus binder, a medication that lowers your phosphorus levels.

Reduce your intake of potassium, as this mineral is essential to the proper functioning of your muscles and nerves. However, when you have, your body cannot remove additional potassium. It can cause serious heart problems if you have too much of it in your blood. Numerous fruits and vegetables, including bananas, potatoes, avocados, oranges, cooked broccoli, raw carrots, greens (with the exception of kale), tomatoes, and melons, contain potassium.

Your blood potassium levels may be affected by these foods. If you need to cut back on this mineral in your diet, your doctor will let you know. If this is the case, they might suggest trying low-potassium foods like:
Cranberries and cranberry juice Strawberries, blueberries, and raspberries Plums Pineapples Peaches Cabbage Boiling cauliflower Asparagus Beans (green or wax) Celery Cucumber as your condition deteriorates, you may need to make additional dietary adjustments.

This may necessitate reducing your intake of foods high in protein, particularly animal protein. Dairy products, seafood, and meats are examples of these. You might also require more iron. Discuss with your doctor the foods that contain iron when you have to manage your chronic kidney disease, you may need to alter your diet.

Develop a meal plan with a registered dietitian that includes foods you enjoy while preserving your kidney health. The means underneath will assist you with eating right as you deal with your kidney infection. The initial three stages (1-3) are significant for all individuals with kidney infection. As your kidney function declines, the final two steps (steps 4-5) may become more significant.

The first steps toward healthy eating Step Step 1: Why should you select and prepare foods with less sodium and salt? to aid in blood pressure control. Your daily sodium intake should not exceed 2,300 milligrams. Buy fresh food frequently. Many prepared or packaged foods that you buy at the supermarket or in restaurants contain sodium, which is a component of salt.

Instead of consuming high-sodium canned foods, "fast" foods, frozen dinners, and prepared meals, cook from scratch. You are in charge of what goes into your food when you make it yourself.
Salt can be substituted for spices, herbs, and seasonings devoid of sodium. On the Nutrition Facts label of food packages, look for sodium. A daily value of 20% or more indicates that the food contains a lot of sodium.

Try frozen dinners and other convenience foods in lower-sodium versions.
Before eating, rinse canned meats, fish, beans, and vegetables with water.
Look for words like salt-free or sodium-free on food labels; or zero, very little, or no sodium or salt; or lightly salted or unsalted.

Step 2: Why should you consume the right kinds and amounts of protein? to aid in renal protection. Your body makes waste when it uses protein. This waste is removed by your kidneys. Your kidneys may have to work harder when you consume more protein than you need. Eat protein foods in small quantities.

Both animal and plant foods contain protein. The majority consume both types of protein. Discuss

with your dietitian how to select the appropriate
protein food combinations for you.
Foods with animal protein:
A cooked serving of chicken, fish, meat, eggs, or
dairy weighs about 2 to 3 ounces, or about the size
of a deck of cards. 12 cup of milk, 1 slice of cheese,
or 1 cup of yogurt constitute a dairy food portion.

Plant-Protein Food Sources:

Beans, nuts, grains, and grains make up about 12
cups and 14 cups, respectively, when cooked. One
slice of bread constitutes a portion, and one cup of
cooked rice or noodles constitutes a portion.

Step 3: Why should you choose heart-healthy foods?
to aid in the prevention of fat accumulation in the
kidneys, heart, and blood vessels.
Instead of deep frying, you can grill, broil, bake,
roast, or stir-fry your food. Instead
of butter, use nonstick cooking spray or a small
amount of olive oil.

Before eating, remove the skin and fat from poultry
and meat. Attempt to restrict soaked and trans fats.
Peruse the food mark.

Heart-Protecting Foods:

Low-fat or fat-free milk, yogurt, and cheese are the
next steps in a healthy diet. As your kidney function
declines, you may need to eat less phosphorus and
potassium-rich foods. Lean cuts of meat like loin
and round poultry without the skin.

Your blood phosphorus and potassium levels will be tested in a lab by your doctor, and you can work with your dietitian to change your meal plan. The NIDDK health topic Nutrition for Advanced Chronic Kidney Disease offers additional details.

Step 4: Why choose beverages and foods low in phosphorus? to aid in the defense of your blood vessels and bones. Phosphorus can build up in the blood when you have. Calcium is taken out of your bones by too much phosphorus in your blood, making your bones thin, weak, and more likely to break. Elevated degrees of phosphorus in your blood can likewise cause bothersome skin, and bone and joint torment.

Food sources Lower in Phosphorus

- New products of the soil
- Breads, pasta, rice
- Rice milk (not improved)
- Corn and rice grains
- Light-shaded soft drinks/pop, for example, lemon-lime or custom made chilled tea

Food sources Higher in Phosphorus

- Meat, poultry, fish
- Grain cereals and oats
- Dairy food sources
- Beans, lentils, nut
- Dull shaded soft drinks/pop, fruit juice, a few packaged or canned chilled teas that have added phosphorus

Many bundled food varieties have added phosphorus. On ingredient labels, look for phosphorus or words that end in "PHOS." Phosphorus may be added to fresh meat, poultry, and deli meats. You can get assistance selecting fresh meats without phosphorus from the butcher.

To reduce the amount of phosphorus in your blood, your doctor may suggest that you take a phosphate binder with your meals. A medicine known as a phosphate binder binds or absorbs phosphorus in the stomach like a sponge. The phosphorus does not enter your blood because it is bound. Instead, the phosphorus is eliminated from your body through stool.

Step 5: Why should you choose foods high in
potassium? to ensure that your nerves and muscles
function properlyl. Blood potassium levels that are
either too high or too low can cause issues.
Potassium can build up in the blood due to damaged
kidneys, which can lead to serious heart issues.

 If you need to lower your potassium level, your
choices for food and drink can help.
Potassium levels can be very high in salt substitutes.
Read the label on the ingredient. The use of salt
substitutes should be discussed with your provider.
Before eating, drain canned vegetables and fruits.

Foods with less potassium include apples, peaches,
carrots, green beans, white bread, pasta, white rice,
rice milk that hasnt been enriched, cooked rice and
wheat cereals, grits, and apple, grape, or cranberry
juice. Foods with more potassium include bananas,
orange juice, potatoes, tomatoes, brown and wild
rice, bran cereals, dairy products, whole-wheat
bread, pasta, beans, and nuts. The medicines you
take may be changed by your doctor.

Chapter 4

The Advantages and Side Effects of Baking Soda/ Sodium Bicarbonate

Baking soda is more than just a cookie ingredient. It can also help you get rid of stains on your teeth and soothe a sore throat. When you need to make a batch of cookies for your family, you probably keep a box of baking soda in the back of your fridge.

You might have taken it when your stomach hurt or cleaned your clothing with it, as well. Baking soda and vinegar might have even been used together in a school science project in the past. Baking soda is a common household item; however, how much do you actually know about this ingredient that seems to be simple?

What Baking Soda May Do for Your Health

Traditionally, due to its ability to neutralize stomach acid, baking soda is a well-liked antacid for treating heartburn and indigestion. For heartburn relief, mix 12 teaspoon (tsp) with 2 cups of water. A disclaimer, however: Baking soda contains a lot of sodium. There are 630 milligrams (mg) of sodium in just 12 teaspoons.

Considering that the Dietary Guidelines for Americans of the United States of America recommend a daily sodium intake of no more than 2,300 mg, 12 teaspoon of baking soda will provide approximately one quarter of that amount.

Before using baking soda to treat heartburn or indigestion, you should talk to your doctor or pharmacist because it may interact with some medications, you shouldnt use baking soda or sodium bicarbonate for more than two weeks without getting permission from your doctor.

According to some intriguing research findings, using baking soda may help you exercise more effectively. Baking soda can improve athletic performance in a variety of sports and exercises, according to a review published in 2021 by the International Society of Sports Nutrition. The authors suggested taking 300 mg of baking soda per kilogram of body weight 60 to 180 minutes before exercise or competition for optimal performance.

In the future, baking soda may also serve as an effective weapon against autoimmune conditions. When consumed, the antacid effect of baking soda may assist in changing the bodys pro-inflammatory immune cells into those that fight inflammation, which may one day be helpful in disease treatment.

What Baking Soda Cant Do for Your Health

Baking soda is one of those ingredients that some people claim can treat a variety of health issues. However, in reality, there is insufficient research to support significant claims, such as the idea that it is a cancer treatment. Baking soda was found to possibly improve the bodys response to cancer therapy in at least one mouse study. A 2020 survey found that a 5 percent sodium bicarbonate arrangement might have anticancer impacts when applied to growths locally in mix with customary disease drugs.

However, this does not mean that a cancer patient can treat their condition at home or avoid conventional therapies. To fully investigate the effects of baking soda on cancer, larger clinical trials in humans are required. This research is still in its early stages.

Can Baking Soda Aid In Weight Loss?

There are no studies that show baking soda can help your body burn more fat or speed up your metabolism. It might assist you in getting more out of your workout. However, there are so many factors that influence the relationship between exercise and weight loss that you cannot expect this to have a significant impact. Additionally, due to its high sodium content, baking soda may cause bloating if consumed excessively.

What Surprising Uses Can Be Found For Baking Soda?

Theres a good reason why baking soda is regarded as a versatile product. Here are just a few of its many applications.

As a Produce Wash Dont waste your money on fancy, expensive produce washes. A basic baking pop and water douse for 12 to 15 minutes is sufficient to eliminate 80 and 96 percent of specific pesticides from apples better than faucet water alone or fade. Baking soda aids in the breakdown of some pesticides, allowing them to be washed away.

As a Natural Cleaner A nonabrasive, effective cleaner that can be made with baking soda and water is Use case: to clean the inside of a refrigerator of old food crumbs. You can also clean your bathtub, sink, and shower curtain with baking soda and hot water, clean your pipes, and remove scuff marks from floors. Additionally, keep in mind that it is an excellent deodorizer. After putting baking soda on a carpet, let it sit for a while before vacuuming it, and the bad smell will go away.

To Safely Clean Pots and Pans, the American Cleaning Institute suggests adding baking soda to the pan, filling it with hot water, and soaking it for 15 to 30 minutes if cooked food remains stuck to the pan. The baking soda will assist in lifting the browned food fragments.

To freshen clothes without the chemicals of other products, add 12 cups of baking soda to the rinse cycle. For occasional episodes of heartburn, mix 12 teaspoons with 12 cups of water and drink. The acid will be neutralized by the alkaline baking soda.

- Take Care of Bug Bites

- Do you know how annoying itchy bug bites can be? you can find relief by applying a paste of baking soda to the bite several times a day (mix baking soda with a little water until you get the right consistency).

- Morning Sickness: The stomach acid produced by vomiting can damage your tooth enamel in addition to causing discomfort. Rinse your mouth with 1 teaspoon of baking soda and water if you experience frequent or occasional vomiting. When illness, such as food poisoning, is causing vomiting, you can also do this.

- ☐ Treat Nail Infections: Baking soda has antifungal properties, so if you have a mild infection, you might want to try a soak in water and baking soda.

- ☐ Ease Inconvenience During Malignant growth

Therapy Rinsing your mouth with a mix of baking pop, salt, and water can assist with facilitating throat uneasiness brought about by radiation or chemotherapy. Additionally, this mixture may aid in the prevention of mouth sores becoming infected.

Make sure to swallow the solution instead of gargling it. Before using any mouth rinses, the American Cancer Society advises consulting your cancer care team because they may occasionally be harmful or aggravate mouth sores.

Baking Sodas Side Effects And Health Risks

There are a few issues to keep in mind if you take too much of it. If you use baking soda and an acid to whiten your teeth at home, this can wear away the enamel over time.

Baking soda can also cause overconsumption due to its high sodium content

An over-burden of sodium can cause spewing and the runs, as well as additional difficult issues like seizures and kidney disappointment. If it produces too much gas when used as an antacid, it can actually exacerbate gastrointestinal issues. Alarmingly, in uncommon examples, taking it in the wake of eating a huge dinner can cause a stomach crack. Stick with safer products like Tums, which are recommended by the National Capital Poison Center. Lastly, if you have high blood pressure, you should consult your doctor before taking it due to its sodium content.

Chapter 5

The power of turmeric, ginger root, activated Charcoal 101: Functions, Benefits, and Dangers

There are a lot of detox supplements out there, and they all say they do one thing: get rid of harmful toxins in the body. The most recent "detoxifying" supplement of choice is activated charcoal, which are the material found in water filtration systems.

People who are otherwise healthy are now taking activated charcoal supplements in the hopes of detoxifying their bodies and treating a variety of ailments, such as diarrhea, gas, kidney problems, hangovers, and yellowed teeth. Activated charcoal was once primarily used in emergency rooms to treat poisonings and overdoses.

In the same way as other enhancements, enacted charcoal is engaging in light of the fact that its not difficult to purchase (no remedy required), fast to take, and it, quote-unquote; helps the body eliminate toxins, which is appealing. Indeed, studies show that supplement use is up tenfold in recent years.

However, supplements alone are not enough to quell the fervor for activated charcoal; It is being added to toothpaste, skin care products, detox drinks, cocktails, and even ice cream. However, in 2018, activated charcoal was outlawed in food and beverages in New York.

To summarize, activated charcoal is a trendy supplement and ingredient. However, there are a few things you should be aware of before jumping on the bandwagon.

How Does Activated Charcoal Work and What Is It?

The charcoal bricks you use to grill food are not the same thing as activated charcoal. It is a black, odorless powder made from carbon-based materials like sawdust, coconut shells, or peat that have been "activated," or heated to make them more porous, at high temperatures.

Should a Detox Cleanse Be Tried?

Activated charcoal can bind toxic substances in the intestines and prevent their absorption into the body when consumed. Some charcoal preparations have a surface area that is nearly one-third the size of a large football field, according to a 2015 review of clinical and animal studies.

Adsorption (attraction of atoms, ions, or molecules from a gas or liquid to a solid surface) of chemicals and toxins is enhanced by this size. The toxins are eliminated through your feces once activated charcoal has trapped them.

The Potential Health Benefits of Activated Charcoal

Activated charcoal proponents tout the ingredients ability to effectively cleanse the body. A few of its potential health benefits are listed below.

Activated charcoal can be used to treat poisoning and drug overdose in a clinical setting because it can trap toxins in the gut, making it useful in emergency situations. In point of fact, activated charcoal is probably beneficial for only that one use. In 1811, activated charcoal was first reported to be used to treat poisonings, but its use declined over time.

When given right away, activated charcoal is most helpful in cases of drug overdose and poisoning. A 2005 position paper says that volunteers who took at least 50 grams (g) of activated charcoal 30 minutes after taking a poison reduced absorption by an average of 47%, based on data from 48 comparisons involving 26 drugs. However, the majority of comparisons utilized small sample sizes, typically ranging from six to ten volunteers.

The majority of the toxin has probably already been absorbed or moved into the intestine because many people dont show symptoms until at least two hours later. However, activated charcoal may assist in reducing the final amount absorbed if digestion has slowed. However, activated charcoal is ineffective for poisonings involving alkalis, strong acids, petroleum products, or alcohols, and should only be used in exceptional circumstances in cases of poisoning and overdose.

May Assist with Treating Wounds

The exploration on what actuated charcoal might mean for wound recuperating might guarantee. For instance, a 2016 study found that people with chronic venous leg ulcers healed faster with carbon cloths carbon is another name for activated charcoal than with other antimicrobial dressings.

 In a similar vein, a study conducted in 2022 found that wounds covered with carbon cloths shrinked more rapidly than wounds covered with a standard silver foam dressing. Yet, enacted charcoal probably doesnt assist with bedsore recuperating, notwithstanding.

May Support Kidney Function

A 2015 review found that activated charcoal may aid in the removal of waste products like urea from the kidneys. This would be beneficial to people with chronic kidney disease, who are unable to remove these waste products as effectively as people with healthy kidneys.

In a small 2010 study, taking 30 g of activated charcoal per day in conjunction with a low-protein diet for ten months led to a significant drop in blood urea and creatinine levels in older people with end-stage renal disease. Keep in mind that this study only had nine participants, so dont take these results too seriously right away).

A low-protein diet may be suggested by your healthcare team if you have kidney disease. Before doctors recommend activated charcoal for supporting kidney function, additional research is required once more.

May Help Reduce Excessive Gas

According to research, activated charcoal may alleviate excess gas. In a small 2003 study, men with and without excessive gas found that activated charcoal effectively reduced bloating and gas. A 2017 observational study found that after 10 days, people with small intestinal bowel overgrowth (SIBO) had 25% less gas when they used activated charcoal and simethicone (Alka-Seltzer is one brand). Greater gas production is linked to SIBO.

However, those who took the antibiotic metronidazole (Flagyl) experienced even better outcomes, with a 67% decrease in gas production. However, a limitation of this study is that participants self-reported their gas incidents in a diary for three days before and after treatment. This makes it difficult to determine whether incidents were accurately reported, and three days is a short time period.

The Best Home Remedies for Bloating and Gas

A panel from the European Food Safety Authority decided that there was enough proof to help the utilization of initiated charcoal for over the top gas.

They recommend taking at least 1 g of the substance approximately 30 minutes prior to eating and 1 g of the substance immediately after eating.

It is essential to keep in mind that the Food and Drug Administration (FDA) of the United States does not regulate any supplement, including activated charcoal, in the same manner that it regulates medical drugs.

May Aid In Diarrhea Treatment And Prevention

Activated charcoal holds toxins in the intestine, it may prevent drugs and bacteria that cause diarrhea from being absorbed into the body. In fact, a 2017 review says that activated charcoal is a good option for treating diarrhea, especially since the supplement has few side effects compared to other antidiarrheal treatments.

However, activated charcoal has not been shown to alleviate diarrhea, according to the Mayo Clinic. To determine whether activated charcoal is effective in treating and preventing diarrhea, additional research is required.

The Secondary effects and Expected Dangers of Utilizing Enacted Charcoal

As a rule, initiated charcoal might be ok for incidental use, yet proceed cautiously, specialists say. A seven-year observational study that was published in 2010 found that adverse reactions to active charcoal are uncommon. However, this study only looked at the use of activated charcoal in hospitals, not as a common household remedy.

May Affect Gut Health

 One of the risks of taking activated charcoal outside of a clinical setting is that the supplement may also remove important nutrients from the digestive tract in the process of trapping and eliminating "toxins." According to a 2015 review, that could disrupt the balance of gut bacteria and pose health risks. On the other hand, it may slow down or stop the absorption of medications. Additionally, activated charcoal may result in undesirable side effects such as vomiting, constipation, and nausea.

May Damage Your Teeth

Notwithstanding the dangers of ingesting enacted charcoal, there are additionally gambles related with utilizing it to clean or brighten your teeth. A 2017 review reveals that these claims about activated charcoals oral detoxification and antibacterial, antifungal, and antiviral properties are not supported by sufficient evidence.

In addition, the reviews three studies reported negative outcomes such as an increase in caries and enamel abrasion, both of which can lead to cavities. The authors advise dentists to advise patients against using charcoal and products with charcoal as a component.

Activated charcoal is also being added to skin-care products by beauty companies. More research is needed to find out how it affects the skin. In a 2017 paper, researchers who used activated charcoal in a skin care product claimed that the product helped fight acne by drawing bacteria, dirt, and other small particles to the surface of the skin.

However, since these claims have not been tested on humans, it is unknown whether activated charcoal has any skin-care benefits. The dangers are also a mystery.

Impacts Are Hazy When Charcoal Is Ingested for Headaches or Different Issues

Theres no exploration to prove the advantages of adding actuated charcoal to food varieties, by the same token. Although black hamburger buns and ice cream may appear cool, it is uncertain whether all that activated charcoal is actually beneficial to your body. In addition, the effects of using activated charcoal to treat or prevent a hangover are also unknown.

 The majority of this research was done decades ago, and the U.S. National Library of Medicine says that the body doesnt seem to be good at trapping activated charcoal, so it probably wont help your aches and pains before or after a night of indulgence.

Is Activated Charcoal Worth Trying?

Although activated charcoal may be an effective detoxifier in some situations, particularly in acute poisonings, the answer to the question of whether it can assist with diarrhea, gas, kidney issues, cosmetic issues, and numerous other benefits is still unknown. Activated charcoal should not be used to treat poisonings or overdoses on your own either.

If you want to give activated charcoal a try, you should do so with the help of a doctor, especially if you are already taking other medications. If the supplement is suitable for your health objectives, your doctor can collaborate with you to determine the appropriate dosage and frequency. Even though activated charcoal has not been linked to birth defects or other health issues in infants, you should still consult your doctor before taking it if you are pregnant or breastfeeding.

For centuries, migraines, chronic inflammation, fatigue, and other conditions have been treated with ginger and turmeric. Ginger and turmeric are two of the most broadly concentrated on fixings in natural medication.

In addition, they have been used to reduce nausea, improve immune function, and alleviate pain in order to protect against illness and infection. The flowering plants ginger and turmeric are both widely used in natural medicine.

Ginger, or Zingiber officinale, comes from Southeast Asia and has been used for a long time as a natural remedy for a variety of health problems.

Gingerol, a chemical that is thought to have potent anti-inflammatory and antioxidant properties, is one of the phenolic compounds that make up the majority of its medicinal properties.
Curcuma longa, also known as turmeric, is a member of the same plant family and is frequently used as a spice in Indian cuisine.

Curcumin, a chemical found in it, has been shown to help treat and prevent a number of chronic conditions. Ginger and turmeric can be eaten whole, ground, or dried, and they can be added to a variety of dishes. Additionally, they are available as supplements.

Studies have shown that both ginger and turmeric can assist in reducing sickness and pain, despite the lack of evidence regarding their effects when used together. reducing sickness and pain.

Reduce inflammation: It is believed that chronic inflammation is a major contributor to the development of diseases such as diabetes, cancer, and heart disease.
It also has the potential to exacerbate the symptoms of autoimmune diseases like rheumatoid arthritis and inflammatory bowel disease.

Ginger and turmeric have strong mitigating properties, which could assist with diminishing agony and safeguard against sickness. One study of 120 people with osteoarthritis found that taking one gram of ginger extract per day for three months effectively reduced inflammation and nitric oxide levels, a molecule that is crucial to the inflammatory process.

In a similar vein, a review of nine studies revealed that taking 1–3 grams of ginger daily for six to twelve weeks reduced levels of the inflammatory marker C-reactive protein (CRP).

Turmeric extract, on the other hand, has been shown in human and test tube studies to reduce a number of inflammation markers, with some studies suggesting that it may be as effective as ibuprofen and aspirin.

Turmeric supplementation may also lower CRP, interleukin-6 (IL-6), and malondialdehyde (MDA) levels, all of which are used to measure body inflammation, according to a 15-study review.

- Curcumin and ginger have both been studied for their capacity to alleviate persistent pain

- Curcumin, the active ingredient in turmeric, is particularly effective at relieving arthritis-related pain, according to studies.

In point of fact, a review of eight studies revealed that taking 1,000 mg of curcumin had the same effect on arthritis patients joint pain as taking certain painkillers.

When compared to a placebo, taking 1,500 mg of curcumin daily significantly reduced pain and improved physical function in 40 people with osteoarthritis.

Additionally, it has been demonstrated that ginger can alleviate the chronic pain associated with arthritis and a number of other conditions. For instance, a 5-day study involving 120 women found that taking 500 mg of powdered ginger root three times per day decreased the intensity and duration of menstrual pain.

Another study with 74 participants found that taking 2 grams of ginger for 11 days significantly reduced exercise-induced muscle pain.

Boost immune function Many people take ginger and turmeric at the first sign of a cold or flu in the hope that doing so will help them avoid the symptoms.

Ginger, in particular, may have potent immune-boosting properties, according to some research.

Fresh ginger was found to be effective against the human respiratory syncytial virus which can cause respiratory tract infections in children, adults, and infants, according to one test-tube study. Ginger extract was found to inhibit the growth of a number of respiratory tract pathogens in another test tube study.

A mouse study also found that taking ginger extract reduced symptoms of seasonal allergies like sneezing and blocked the activation of several pro-inflammatory immune cells. In a similar vein, studies in animals and test tubes have demonstrated that curcumin has antiviral properties and can assist in reducing the severity of the influenza A virus.

Inflammation levels can be reduced by both ginger and turmeric, which can help the immune system function better.
However, the majority of studies rely on concentrated doses of turmeric or ginger in test tubes or on animals.

To determine how each can affect human immune health when consumed in normal amounts, additional research is required.
Reduce nausea Ginger has been shown in a number of studies to be an effective natural remedy for calming the stomach and reducing nausea.

One study of 170 women found that taking one gram of ginger powder every day for a week was just as effective as taking a common anti-nausea medication to reduce nausea caused by pregnancy, but it had far fewer side effects.

Additionally, a review of five studies revealed that taking at least one gram of ginger daily could significantly reduce nausea and vomiting following surgery.

Other exploration demonstrates that ginger can diminish queasiness brought about by movement infection, chemotherapy, and certain gastrointestinal problems.

Some studies have found that turmeric may protect against digestive issues caused by chemotherapy, which could help reduce symptoms like nausea, vomiting, and diarrhea. However, more research is needed to evaluate the effects of turmeric on nausea. Ginger and turmeric may help reduce inflammation markers, alleviate chronic pain, reduce nausea, and enhance immune function, according to some studies.

Side effects Ginger and turmeric are considered safe and healthy additions to a well-rounded diet when used in moderation. In any case, a few potential secondary effects should be thought of.
To begin, some studies have shown that high doses of ginger may inhibit blood clotting and interact with blood thinners.

Before taking ginger supplements, people who are taking medications to lower their blood sugar levels should also talk to their doctor about it. In addition, bear in mind that the curcumin content of turmeric powder is only about 3% by weight; consequently, in order to attain the dosage recommended by the majority of studies, you would either need to consume a very large amount of turmeric powder or take a supplement.

Curcumin has been linked to side effects like diarrhea, headaches, and rashes when taken in large quantities. Lastly, although there is a lot of research on the potential health effects of ginger and turmeric, there is little information on how the two may affect health when used together.

Before taking a supplement, check with a doctor, and if you notice any side effects, reduce the dosage. Ginger may lower blood sugar and prevent blood clots. How to use ginger and turmeric There are a variety of ways to incorporate ginger and turmeric into your diet to reap the numerous health benefits that each has to offer, including rashes, headaches, and diarrhea when taken in high doses.

Salad dressings, stir-fries, and sauces made with these two ingredients add flavor and health benefits to your favorite dishes.

In addition, fresh ginger can be added to curries, smoothies, soups, and ginger shots, or brewed into a soothing tea.

On the other hand, using turmeric to brighten up dishes like casseroles, frittatas, dips, and dressings is a great idea.

Additionally available as a supplement, ginger root extract has been shown to be most effective when taken daily at doses of 1,500 to 2,000 mg. A pinch of black pepper, which can help increase your bodys absorption of turmeric by up to 2,000 percent, is ideal. Turmeric supplements can provide a more concentrated dose of curcumin and can be taken twice daily in doses of 500 mg to alleviate pain and inflammation.

Supplements that contain both turmeric and ginger are accessible too, making it simple to get your fix of each in a solitary day to day portion. These supplements can be purchased locally or online. Both ginger and turmeric can be consumed fresh, dried, or as a supplement, making them simple to incorporate into ones diet.

Ginger and turmeric have been shown to have potent effects on nausea, pain, inflammation, and immune function in a number of promising studies. However, there is a lack of evidence regarding the effects of combining the two, and the majority of the research that is available is restricted to studies in test tubes. Having said that, both can be consumed without causing any harm to ones health and can be a healthy addition to a diet that is well-balanced.

Chapter 6

Supplement with antioxidants that can improve renal function

An oxidant is a substance that can take up electrons, while a reductant is a compound that gives up electrons. Oxidation, on the other hand, is a chemical reaction in which a compound gains electrons, while reduction is a chemical process in which electrons are lost.

At the point when an oxidant acquires electrons, it sets off the oxidation of another compound, and while a lessening specialist gives its electrons, it causes the decrease of another substance. As a result, a reduction process always follows an oxidation reaction, and vice versa.

Redox reactions are the names given to these chemical reactions. The biochemical terms "oxidant" and "reductant" should be changed to "prooxidant" and "antioxidant" in cells and tissues, respectively. The ratio of prooxidant to antioxidant agents is known as the redox potential or redox state. Under pathological conditions, this state can shift toward redosis or oxidosis. Oxidation brings about creation of responsive oxygen species (ROS).

ROS are not only necessary for cellular growth and proliferation, but they are also linked to a number of harmful processes.
The interruption of harmony between creation of ROS and cell reinforcement frameworks is named oxidative pressure (operating system). According to this OS paradox, a lot of antioxidants in a cellular environment might scavenge too many reactive oxygen species (ROS) and prevent them from stimulating important biochemical reactions that are necessary for cell homeostasis.

The two-sided disturbance of equilibrium of the redox state to either exorbitant decrease or oxidation brings about injury and harm of the natural frameworks. Endogenous antioxidants (the bodys natural defense mechanisms) and exogenous antioxidants (supplements and food) are the two types of antioxidants. Endogenous antioxidants can be enzymatic or nonenzymatic, and they can be molecules that dissolve in water or fat.

Constant kidney illness is an overall medical condition which has appeared as a pandemic during the previous many years. Traditional risk factors cannot solely account for its rising incidence rates and significant cardiovascular burden. OS is a novel nontraditional risk factor for all-cause and CV mortality in these patients and is thought to be an important pathogenetic mechanism in uremia.

OS is exacerbated in hemodialysis (HD) patients and occurs even in the early stages of augments in tandem with the progression of the disease to end-stage renal disease. Compared to nondialysis uremic patients, ESRD patients on peritoneal dialysis (PD) have a significantly improved OS, but HD patients have a lower OS.

Various mediations have been recommended to improve operating system in dialysis patients. This audit is pointed toward introducing the accessible information in regards to the exogenous organization of cancer prevention agents and their conceivable defensive consequences for renal substitution treatment (RRT) patients.

Renal Substitution Treatment And Operating System

A few variables are embroiled in the pathogenesis of operating system in HD and PD. ESRD patients normally have various comorbidities connected with inordinate creation of prooxidants, similar to hypertension, dyslipidemia, diabetes mellitus (DM), vascular calcification, and advanced age .

ROS production is frequently sparked by chronic inflammation and malnutrition that accompany dialysis patients. Prooxidant formation is also aided by RRT-related factors. White blood cells and platelets are activated, leading to the acute production of reactive oxygen species (ROS) within minutes of the beginning of the HD session, as a result of blood exposure to bioincompatible dialysate, dialyzers, the use of heparin, and the administration of intravenous iron.

The levels of ROS in the bloodstream rise by 14 times during each HD session. Prooxidant formation in PD is caused by the bioincompatibility of PD solutions, which includes high osmolality, elevated lactate levels, low pH, and accumulation of advanced glycation end-products (AGEs). The ultrafiltrate loses a lot of vitamins as a result.

 Patients on RRT are characterized by a significant depletion of antioxidant defense mechanisms, in addition to the formation of prooxidant molecules, for a number of reasons: While treatment with either PD or HD has been linked to a loss of vitamins and trace elements, both the traditional, strict dietary restrictions and the malnutrition that typically accompany ESRD patients are characterized by a lack of fruit and vegetable consumption.

As a result, a low intake of antioxidants like vitamins C, D, and E. Along these lines, it has been speculated that organization of a few exogenous cell reinforcements could shield RRT patients from operating system determined cardiovascular dismalness, irritation, and mortality.

In addition, it was showed that 600 mg/day per operating system treatment with vitamin E for a considerable length of time in HD patients diminished the gamble of operating system prompted CVD.
Vitamin E appears to reduce OS in RRT patients, as evidence mounts.

She analyzed the impact of vitamin E on endogenous cancer prevention agent frameworks and lipid peroxidation status in 46 support HD patients, partitioned in 3 gatherings: 10 untreated individuals, 36 receiving EPO (100 U/kg) three times per week for three months, and 36 receiving a 50 percent lower dosage of EPO and 300 mg/day of oral vitamin E for three months.

When measured by the activities of superoxide dismutase (SOD) and catalase (CAT), those who were treated with the combination of EPO and vitamin E had significantly improved antioxidant status in comparison to the two other groups. In another study, dialysis patients with HD or PD were treated with a low dose of 300 mg of vitamin E taken orally three times per week.

In a placebo-controlled study, 13 PD and 34 HD patients were randomly assigned to receive either 300 mg of vitamin E taken or placebo for 20 weeks. OS status was significantly reduced in HD and PD patients treated with vitamin E. Another study on people with Parkinsons disease found that taking a combination of vitamins E and C prevented the

formation of prooxidants in urine, blood, and
peritoneal fluid when taken orally.

Vitamin E oral intake at a dose of 500-800 mg/day
was also found to have a beneficial antioxidant
effect in three open-label trials on maintenance HD
patients. Omega-3 fatty acids and vitamin E were
the only nutritional interventions that, according to a
meta-analysis of 46 randomized controlled trials,
significantly reduced circulating inflammatory
markers.

Vitamin C (Ascorbic Acid)

During HD therapy, ascorbic acid free radicals are formed and a significant amount of vitamin C is lost, resulting in improved OS. Clermont and co found that ascorbyl free radical formation and a significant drop in plasma vitamin C levels occurred during a dialysis session using a highly biocompatible synthetic membrane.

Additionally, numerous researchers hypothesized that vitamin C supplementation might reduce OS in HD patients because dialysis patients frequently lack the powerful antioxidant vitamin C.In cohorts of stable HD patients, daily oral administration of vitamin C (250 mg) significantly reduced plasma OS biomarkers, whereas only a single high dose of vitamin C (2 g) successfully suppressed OS induced by the HD procedure.

In a group of maintenance HD patients, the combination therapy with daily oral vitamins E (600 mg) and C (200 mg) reduced lipid peroxidation and improved microcirculation. During HD sessions, intravenous vitamin C (1 g) and dialysate enriched with ascorbic acid were used to suppress DNA oxidation in lymphocytes, reduce serum levels of lipid peroxides and AGEs, and inhibit the formation and accumulation of free radicals.

Several researchers disagreed with these findings, stating that vitamin C did not reduce OS, while two studies found that vitamin C supplementation increased oxidative activity. In chronic HD patients, both oral vitamin C (1.5 grams) and intravenous vitamin C (480 mg per HD session) triggered an oxidative response.

Although vitamin C deficiency is well-established in Parkinsons disease patients and is associated with increased inflammation, only a small number of researchers investigated the antioxidant potential of vitamin C supplementation. Demonstrated that low-dose ascorbic acid intake may be beneficial and that vitamin C levels are strongly and independently correlated with OS status in PD patients.

The term "vitamin B family" refers to a group of similar essential nutrients. Folic acid and vitamin B are two examples. The groups most active compounds are vitamin B1 (thiamin), vitamin B6 (pyridoxine), vitamin B12 (cobalamin), and vitamin B9 (folic acid). Folic acid is a component of the vitamin B complex that is necessary for the synthesis of DNA and metabolism of amino acids. Folic acid, along with vitamins B6 and B12, have long been used to lower homocysteine levels in the blood, a biomarker of protein oxidation linked to cardiovascular disease.

Folic Acid And Vitamin B12

Supplementation significantly reduces the genomic damage in the lymphocytes of chronic HD patients in vitro. A growing body of evidence suggests that B6 is a powerful inhibitor of advanced glycation and lipoperoxidation processes. It does this by directly scavenging and neutralizing free radicals that are produced during lipid oxidation. Pyridoxamine supplementation prevented renal function decline and improved albuminuria in diabetic rats.

A daily oral intake of pyridoxamine (doses ranged from 100 to 500 mg) for six months resulted in significant preservation of renal function and decreased urinary levels of inflammatory cytokines, according to two multicenter placebo-controlled trials in diabetic nephropathy patients.

Dialysis patients with secondary hyperparathyroidism exhibit accelerated OS and inflammation. Vitamin D analogs Wu and co. conducted a study to determine how 25 stable HD patients oxidation and inflammatory status were affected by vitamin D analogues, which are currently the first-line treatment for SHP.

Thats what the creators exhibited, contrasted with benchmark, following a 16-week treatment with calcitriol, a few serum incendiary and operating system biomarkers were fundamentally smothered. After a three-month intravenous treatment with selective vitamin D receptor activators, serum levels of several OS and inflammatory biomarkers significantly decreased.

In PD patients, the information with respect with the impact of vitamin D analogs on operating system are scant and just got from trial studies. In vitro as well as in vivo examinations in mice showed that the dynamic type of vitamin D repressed collection of free revolutionaries and glycoxidation and subsequently could safeguard the peritoneum homeostasis, through improvement of operating system status.

OS improvement may be one of vitamin Ds pleotropic effects on dialysis patients. Since there are currently very few data on this, supplementation should not be based on its antioxidant properties.

Green Tea

Green tea is made out of nutrients, minerals, and catechins-notable and viable free extreme scroungers. Green tea has been suggested to prevent atheromatosis and cardiovascular disease in both the general population and dialysis patients in addition to its antioxidant properties.

A meta-analysis of 31 studies found weak evidence that daily consumption of 600-1500 milliliters of green tea can reduce lipid oxidation, increase TAC, and possibly prevent cardiovascular disease.

Due to the fact that dialysis and high OS are states of accelerated oxidation, it seemed reasonable to hypothesize that green tea might be beneficial to these patients. These beneficial effects of green tea were more pronounced in patients exposed to high OS.

A few examinations in creature models with different kinds of renal harm (diabetic nephropathy, lupus nephritis, glomerulonephritis, and urethral hindrance) proposed that green tea treatment could safeguard against protein and lipid oxidation, forestall atherosclerosis, and protect renal capability

.

There are few human studies on dialysis patients who consume green tea. Park and co. divided forty patients on chronic dialysis into two groups: for four weeks, those who consumed a high dose of green tea (5 g/day) and those who consumed equal amounts of water found that green tea significantly improved endothelial function by suppressing OS and inflammation.

In a similar vein, catechins were found to be more effective antioxidant scavengers than vitamin C in the same cohort reported that 20 stable chronic HD patients received 1 g of green tea daily for six months, resulting in an improvement in cardiac function (as measured by a decrease in left ventricular mass) and a significant decrease in OS and inflammatory state.

Green teas anti-inflammatory and antioxidant properties may also have an antiatherogenic protective effect in these high-risk patients, according to the studys authors. There is some proof that green tea utilization could offer assurance from atherosclerosis and CVD and improve operating system in dialysis patients.

However, the data is insufficient to reach a definitive conclusion due to its extremely limited nature. In order to determine its antioxidant and antiatherogenic effects on dialysis patients, additional large-scale cohort studies are needed because there are no significant side effects.

10 Kidney-Friendly Antioxidant Foods

Not only are fresh, vibrant, and kidney-friendly fruits and vegetables beneficial, They are beneficial to individuals with chronic kidney disease. Strong compounds known as antioxidants, which can be found in some foods, may help protect you from cancer, heart disease, Alzheimers, and Parkinsons diseases.

Free radicals, the normal but harmful byproducts produced when your body produces energy, fights infection, or is exposed to toxins, are neutralized by antioxidants. Cancer prevention agent nutrients A, C and E accessible in supplement structure can be hurtful to individuals on dialysis, however many take a renal nutrient enhancement that contains 60-100 mg of L-ascorbic acid each day as suggested by their PCP.
For the kidney diet, here are ten colorful foods high in antioxidants.

Cranberries

Cranberries give sweet breads, muffins, and other dishes like Easy Cranberry Salad a distinctive zing. Appreciate dried cranberries sprinkled on a plate of mixed greens or all alone as a tidbit. You can also consume cranberry juice or a cocktail made with cranberry juice.

Crude cranberries in a 1/2 cup portion provide 1 mg of sodium, 40 mg of potassium, and 6 mg of phosphorus.

3 mg of sodium, 22 mg of potassium, and 3 mg of phosphorus per 1/2 cup serving of mixed cranberry juice.
Dried cranberries, 1/2 cup serving, contain 2 mg of sodium, 24 mg of potassium, and 5 mg of phosphorus.

Black plums

It contain more antioxidants than red plums. Plums should feel fairly firm to slightly supple. You can use plums in smoothies, purée them for Quick Fruit Sorbet, or make Old-Fashioned Plum Cake by pitting and freezing them.
1 medium plum = 0 mg sodium, 104 mg potassium, 11 mg phosphorus

Blueberries

They are a common ingredient in blueberry muffins and pancakes. You can use them in smoothies or a Blueberry Peach Crisp if you buy them frozen. Take pleasure in a bowl of fresh blueberries when they are in season.

Fresh blueberries contain 4 mg sodium, 65 mg potassium, and 7 mg phosphorus per 1/2 cup serving.

Raspberry and blackberry fruits

Fresh berries may be added to cereal or oatmeal, frozen berries can be used in smoothies, or baked berries can be used in pies like More Mommas Blackberry Mountain Pie. To enhance the flavor of meats, use berries in unexpected ways, like in this recipe for Raspberry Wings.
1 mg of sodium, 117 mg of potassium, and 16 mg of phosphorus are found in 1 cup of blackberries; 0 mg of sodium, 93 mg of potassium, and 17 mg of phosphorus are found in 1 cup of raspberries.

Garlic

Garlic is a tiny antioxidant powerhouse that can be used in Garlic Chicken with Balsamic Vinegar or other savory dishes. It can be purchased fresh, bottled, minced, or powdered. A head of garlic can be roasted to soften its flavor and make a delicious spread for bread.

1 clove of garlic contains 4 mg phosphorus, 12 mg sodium, and 1 mg potassium.

Apples

Apple with the peel on have more antioxidants, so wash them, chop them, and add them to chicken or tuna salad for a delicious snack. They can also be baked in apple crisp, cobbler, or pie.
1 medium, skin-on apple has zero sodium, 158 mg of potassium, and 10 mg of phosphorus.

Strawberries

For a summertime dessert, combine fresh strawberries with angel food cake and whipped topping or add them to cereal and salads. Smoothies and desserts like Strawberry Mousse and Red, White, and Blue Salad use frozen or fresh strawberries to boost their antioxidant power.

Fresh strawberries, 1/2 cup (5 medium), contain 1 mg sodium, 120 mg potassium, and 13 mg phosphorus. Red Bell Peppers As a snack, eat red bell peppers raw with a dip or add them to tuna or chicken salad and serve it on bread or crackers.

Peppers can be roasted and put on sandwiches, chopped up for an omelet, or added to kabobs cooked on the grill.

Red bell pepper

It contains 1 mg sodium, 88 mg potassium, and 10 mg phosphorus per 1/2 cup serving. Red cabbage Cooked cabbage has more antioxidants per ounce than raw cabbage. Red cabbage can be served as a healthy side dish in the microwave, steamed, or boiled. It also works well in main dishes like Turkey.

Cabbage Rolls

Coleslaw or cabbage salad can be made with raw red cabbage.
A serving of cooked red cabbage contains 21 mg of sodium, 197 mg of potassium, and 25 mg of phosphorus. A serving of raw shredded red cabbage contains 9 mg of sodium, 85 mg of potassium, and 11 mg of phosphorus.

Red leaf lettuce

The red or purple variety that recognizes red leaf lettuce from the conventional kind contains limited quantities of the strong cell reinforcements beta-carotene and lutein. For the best flavor, wash the leaves carefully and use within three days. Make Chicken Lettuce Wraps to give it a try.
1 leaf of red leaf lettuce = 4 mg sodium, 32 mg potassium, 5 mg phosphorus.

However, Spices like cinnamon, curry powder, pepper, oregano, and turmeric add more than just flavor to food; Even in small quantities, these concentrated antioxidant sources can contribute to your daily intake.

Chapter 7

How vitamin D and vitamin B6 can help the kidneys function better

Chronic kidney disease has been identified as a major global health issue due to its increased risk of cardiovascular and total morbidity and mortality. Lack of vitamin D or inadequacy is normal in patients with , and serum levels of vitamin D seem to have a converse connection with kidney capability. There is mounting evidence to suggest that patients with may suffer from vitamin D deficiency, which may also be associated with worsening renal function and rising rates of morbidity and mortality.

In animal models, recent studies have shown that treatment with active vitamin D or its analogues can reduce fibrosis, apoptosis, and inflammation, thereby reducing renal injury; In patients with, this treatment also reduces proteinuria and mortality. In addition to its pleiotropic effects on extra-mineral metabolism, vitamin D treatment has renoprotective effects that go far beyond its traditional role in maintaining bone and mineral metabolism.

The altered metabolism of vitamin D in kidney disease and the potential renoprotective mechanisms discovered in clinical and experimental studies are the subjects of this review. The effects of vitamin D treatment on clinical outcomes are also the subject of discussion.
A photochemical process produces vitamin D, a steroid prohormone, in the skin from cholesterol-derived precursors (such as 7-dehydrocholesterol).

 Alternately, vitamin D can be obtained from fish oils, fortificd dairy products, mushrooms, and other dietary sources. There are two naturally occurring, inactive forms of vitamin D: vitamin D3 (cholecalciferol), which comes from animal skin and products, and vitamin D2 (ergocalciferol), which doesnt come from animals, are the two forms of vitamin D.

Through two hydroxylation steps, the liver and kidney transform these inactive forms into their biologically active forms. The livers metabolism to produce 25-hydroxyvitamin D (25(OH)D) is the first step in the vitamin D metabolic activation process.

Since this is the primary form of vitamin D that circulates and stores, it is used as a measure of vitamin D levels.

However, extrarenal cells and tissues, such as the prostate, breasts, colon, lungs, pancreatic cells, monocytes, endothelial cells, vascular smooth muscle cells, osteoblasts, and parathyroid cells, have all been found to contain this enzyme. At these sites, this extra-renal-produced 1,25(OH)2D primarily functions as an autocrine or paracrine factor and may be involved in a variety of non-classical vitamin D actions.

Vitamin D metabolism and regulation of its circulating levels are heavily reliant on the kidney. As a result, vitamin D deficiency may result from impaired renal function, as has been observed in patients with Over time.

However, 1,25(OH)2D levels drop even when GFR decreases only slightly, suggesting that vitamin D metabolite deficiency in kidney disease may be caused by a different mechanism. The receptor megalin absorbs the 25(OH)D that is bound to its carrier, the vitamin D-binding protein, into the proximal tubules after passing through the glomerulus.

Megalin is an endocytic receptor that also helps the renal tubule reabsorb albumin and other proteins with low molecular weights. Interestingly, despite adequate substrate delivery to the kidney proximal tubules, megalin knockout mice develop low molecular weight proteinuria and lose a lot of vitamin D/vitamin D binding protein in their urine, leading to severe vitamin D deficiency and bone disease. The vitamin D receptor (VDR) complex and active vitamin D induce renal megalin. As a result, decreased megalin may cause vitamin D deficiency, resulting in a vicious cycle for active vitamin D production and 25(OH)D uptake.

The rise in fibroblast growth factor 23 (FGF-23) levels, which can directly suppress the activity and expression of 1-hydroxylase, is another important factor that can lead to low vitamin D status during kidney disease. With a decrease in GFR and an increase in phosphate, serum levels of FGF-23 rise. In addition, renal 1-hydroxylase activity and messenger ribonucleic acid (mRNA) expression are decreased by phosphate intake, independent of changes in calcium and parathyroid hormone (PTH) levels. Therefore, the suppressed activation of 1-hydroxylase, which decreases the levels of 1,25(OH)2D, and the upregulated expression of 24-hydroxylase, which decreases the concentration of circulating 1,25(OH)2D, may be a major mechanism contributing to the suppressed activation of 1-hydroxylase. The activity of 1-hydroxylase may also be inhibited by N-terminally truncated PTH fragments or the progressive retention of uremic toxins, in addition to these factors. Considered to be an important determinant of the progression of cardiovascular and renal diseases, vitamin D deficiency is associated with an increase in proteinuria and inflammation in the kidney.

A few examinations have shown a connection betweens lack of vitamin D and an expanded level of albuminuria . In a recent meta-analysis, active vitamin D therapy with either paricalcitol or calcitriol provided a significant reduction in proteinuria in patients with in addition to current use of RAAS blockade. Additionally, the Vitamin D receptor Activator for Albuminuria Lowering study confirmed that adding 2 g paricalcitol for RAAS blockade reduces albuminuria and blood pressure in patients with diabetic nephropathy. Proteinuria decreased by 16% in patients receiving active vitamin D treatment, whereas it increased by 6% in patients receiving the control treatment, according to that study.

Heart disease has been linked to vitamin D deficiency in both those with the condition and the general population. In experimental models of cardiac hypertrophy, treatment with active vitamin D reduces myocardial hypertrophy and prevents heart failure. The Paricalcitol Capsule Benefits in Renal Failure Induced Cardiac Morbidity study looked at how paricalcitol helped patients with stage 3 and stage 4 left ventricular hypertrophy. The primary endpoint, changes in the left ventricular mass index (LVMI), did not differ significantly between the paricalcitol-treated and control groups. However, the paricalcitol-treated group had fewer cardiovascular-related hospitalizations. In a similar vein, a recent prospective randomized controlled trial demonstrated that patients in stages 3 to 5 receiving oral paricalcitol did not experience an improvement in cardiac function or LVMI after 52 weeks of treatment. Its possible that paricalcitol increased FGF-23 expression, which directly causes cardiomyopathy in animal models, contributed to these findings.

In contrast, there is mounting evidence that patients with are also more likely to die from noncardiovascular causes, such as infections and cancer. Vitamin D levels below 15 ng/mL were associated with a significant increase in noncardiovascular mortality when compared to levels below 30 ng/mL in the NHANES III cohort study of 3,011 patients who were not on dialysis. Additionally, vitamin D regulates the immune system and acts as an anti-inflammatory. Given the high prevalence of, a recent small randomized controlled trial demonstrated that oral cholecalciferol supplementation reduces serum MCP-1 in patients with early progressive loss of kidney function. This condition is associated with significant morbidity and mortality and is a significant global health issue.Finding novel therapeutic agents that can stop the progression of kidney function loss or even improve kidney function has increased interest due to the limitations of traditional pharmacological therapy, such as RAAS blockade and statins, in delaying the progression of kidney injury. In a variety of experimental models by preventing fibrosis, apoptosis, and inflammation during treatment with active vitamin D or its analogues, renoprotective effects are achieved.

Also, predialysis and dialysis patients much of the time experience the ill effects of lack of vitamin D or inadequacy, and serum vitamin D levels have all the earmarks of being contrarily connected with kidney capability. Vitamin D analogues like paricalcitol are emerging as potential treatment options for improving clinical outcomes in hemodialysis patients and patients with advanced kidney disease. These studies show that the traditional function of vitamin D in maintaining bone and mineral metabolism is not the only explanation for the reduction in proteinuria and mortality seen in patients receiving active vitamin D.

However, vitamin D treatment is currently only recommended for patients with moderate hyperparathyroidism, secondary hyperparathyroidism, and vitamin D deficiency. Among the many issues that need to be resolved are testing the various vitamin D analogues, determining whether nutritional vitamin D truly increases survival, and determining whether clinical outcomes vary according to disease-specific vitamin D metabolism. To respond to these inquiries and find the possible renoprotective components of vitamin

D treatment for patients with, further exploration is required.

Vitamin B6, which can be found in food, helps both the metabolism and the nervous system. It is responsible for making synapses like serotonin and dopamine and converting food into energy.
Vitamin B6 is one of the eight B vitamins. This group of vitamins is necessary for the functioning of cells. They support cell health maintenance, blood cell formation, and metabolism.
A water-soluble vitamin that dissolves in water is vitamin B6, also known as pyridoxine. People must consume sufficient amounts of vitamin B6 every day because the body does not store it and excretes any excess in the urine.
This article examines the health benefits and food sources of vitamin B6, in addition to a persons daily requirement for the vitamin. Deficits and supplements are also discussed.

Benefits Of Vitamin B6 For The Body

Vitamin B6 is involved in more than 100 enzyme reactions and performs numerous body functions. Its primary function is to assist the body in converting proteins, fats, and carbohydrates into energy.

Additionally, this vitamin is involved in: Insusceptible framework capability mental health during pregnancy and youth produces synapses like serotonin and dopamine and hemoglobin, which is the oxygen-conveying part of red platelets.

The following sections examine the effects of vitamin B6 on human health.
Brain function Vitamin B6 is needed to make neurotransmitters, which are important chemical messengers in the brain. Additionally, it helps regulate brain energy use.

A lack of vitamin B6 may be linked to cognitive decline and dementia, according to some research. Based on research, studies have shown us that older adults with higher blood levels of vitamin B6 have better memory. In any case, there is lacking proof to propose that taking vitamin B6 supplements further develops discernment or mind-set in dementia patients or non-dementia patients.

Nausea during pregnancy

A review study suggests that taking pyridoxine may reduce mild nausea and vomiting symptoms during pregnancy when compared to a placebo. Additionally, it states that combining pyridoxine and doxylamine may help alleviate symptoms.

Based on the findings of the study, the American Congress of Obstetricians and Gynecologists (ACOG) suggests taking vitamin B6 supplements as a safe over-the-counter remedy for nausea during pregnancy.

Protection from air pollution A 2017 study found that vitamin B6 may help people avoid the negative effects of air pollution by lowering the impact of pollution on the epigenome. The researchers hope that new approaches to halting air pollution-induced epigenetic changes will emerge from their findings.

Vitamin B6 can be tracked down in many food varieties in some structure. A diet that is well-balanced tends to stop the development of deficiencies. Certain medications and medical conditions can result in a deficiency.

Foods containing vitamin B6 include the following:
A cup of chickpeas contains 1.1 milligrams (mg),
which is 65% of the day to day esteem (DV);
3 ounces of beef liver have 0.9 mg, or 53% of the
DV;
3 ounces of yellowfin tuna has 0.9 mg, or 53% of
the DV;
3 ounces of roasted chicken breast contains 0.5 mg,
or 29% of the DV; Potatoes have 0.4 mg per cup, or
25% of the fortified foods, including breakfast
cereals, salmon, turkey, marinara sauce, ground
beef, waffles, bulgur, cottage cheese, squash, rice,
raisins, onion, spinach, and watermelon.

B6 deficiency In the United States, B6 deficiency is
uncommon, but it can happen if a person takes
estrogens, corticosteroids, anticonvulsants, or other
medications or has poor intestinal absorption.

Vitamin B6 deficiency is frequently accompanied by
low levels of other B vitamins like folate and
vitamin B12.
A B6 deficiency can eventually occur as a result of
long-term excessive alcohol consumption, diabetes,
hypothyroidism, or both.

Vitamin B6 deficiency causes the following symptoms and side effects:
A lack of vitamin B6 can occasionally cause symptoms like pellagra, like tingling, numbness, and pain in the hands and feet; anemia; seizures; depression; confusion; and a compromised immune system
Seizures can continue even after anticonvulsant treatment for newborn children with seborrheic dermatitis, glossitis, or cheilosis, which causes irritation and breaking of the lips.

One example of a deficiency that can last a lifetime is peripheral neuropathy.
B6 supplements

Vitamin B6 supplements are consumed by 28-36% of Americans. Supplements can be in form of capsule and tablet forms.
The majority of people, regardless of age, in the United States consume sufficient B6 and do not require supplements.

Low B6 levels are more common in the following groups:
There is no evidence that eating a lot of food with a lot of vitamin B6 has a bad effect on people who

drink a lot of liquor, are overweight, or are pregnant or breastfeeding. However, a body loss movement control and severe, progressive sensory neuropathy have been linked to oral pyridoxine use for 12 to 40 months.

The majority of nutrients should come from food, according to the Dietary Guidelines for Americans for 2015 to 2020. They support utilization of a reasonable eating routine with supplement thick food varieties and a lot of dietary fiber.
Summary: The nervous system and metabolism are both dependent on vitamin B6, a vital vitamin.

Since the body does not store this vitamin, individuals must consume it daily from their diets. The majority of Americans consume enough vitamin B6 through their diets. If not, a doctor might tell you to change your diet or take vitamin B6 supplements.

Chapter 8

How antioxidant teas can help the kidneys function better

Herbal Tea

It benefits People all over the world have been drinking tea for a very good reason for thousands of years. Numerous studies have demonstrated that a variety of teas may strengthen your immune system, reduce inflammation, and even prevent heart disease and cancer. Even though some teas have better health benefits than others, there is a lot of evidence that drinking tea on a regular basis can improve your health over time. Put on your kettle because were going to show you some of the best benefits that are hidden in the most popular teas in the world.

Benefits of White Tea

White tea is made from the Camellia sinensis plant, which is native to China and India and is known for its delicate flavor. It is likewise the most un-handled tea assortment. Due to its high level of antioxidants, research indicates that it may be the most effective cancer fighting tea.

White tea may also be good for your teeth because it has a lot of catechins, tannins, and fluoride, all of which can strengthen teeth, fight plaque, and make them more resistant to sugar and acid. Additionally, this variety contains the least amount of caffeine, making it an excellent option for tea drinkers who wish to limit or avoid caffeine intake.

Similar to white tea, herbal teas, also known as tisanes, contain a blend of herbs, spices, fruits, or other plants in addition to tea leaves. Home grown teas dont contain caffeine, which is the reason theyre known for their quieting properties.
Herbal teas come in a wide variety of flavors and strengths.
The following are some of the most popular herbal teas:

- ☐ Rooibos– Improves blood pressure and circulation, boosts good cholesterol while lowering bad cholesterol, keeps hair strong and skin healthy, and provides allergy relief.
- ☐ Peppermint – Contains menthol, which has the ability to alleviate stomach pain and treat constipation, IBS, and motion sickness.
- ☐ Chamomile Tea – Helps to reduce menstrual pain and muscle spasms. Additionally, this variety of tea helps alleviate migraine and tension headache pain.
- ☐ Hibiscus – Lowers blood pressure and fat levels, improves overall liver health, can starve off cravings for unhealthy sweets, and may prevent the formation of kidney stones

Benefits of Green Tea

Green tea originates from China, where the leaves are processed with heat using a pan-firing or roasting method, and Japan, where the leaves are more commonly steamed.

- Ginger – Helps to combat morning sickness, can be used to treat chronic indigestion, and helps to relieve joint pain caused by osteo. Green tea is astoundingly high in flavonoids that can assist with supporting your heart wellbeing by bringing down terrible cholesterol and lessening blood thickening.

This kind of tea has also been shown in studies to lower total cholesterol, triglycerides, and blood pressure.
Other exploration has found that green tea conceivably affects liver, bosom, prostate and colorectal tumors. Additionally, this variety of tea has been shown to be anti-inflammatory, which contributes to clear and glowing skin.

Matcha, a type of green tea, has gained popularity in recent years. Matcha is a very fine, high-quality powder of green tea made from the whole leaves of tea bushes that are grown in the shade. Since it is the main type of tea where the leaves are ingested, matcha contains significantly more cancer prevention agents that customary green tea. In point of fact, some people have suggested that 10 cups of regular green tea are the same as one cup of matcha.

Benefits of Black Tea

Camellia sinensis, the same plant that is used to make green tea, produces black tea. Black tea, on the other hand, has a darker color and a more complex flavor because the leaves are dried and fermented.

Black tea, unlike many other varieties, contains caffeine, so its important to keep track of how much you drink. Flavonoids that support healthy immune function and combat inflammation are available to you when you sip a cup of black tea. However, the health benefits of black tea are not limited to consumption.

It can be applied to minor cuts, scrapes, and bruises by steaming, cooling, and then pressing to reduce swelling. Additionally, skin rashes and conditions like poison ivy can be alleviated by a black tea bath.

Benefits of Oolong Tea

Oolong tea is a traditional Chinese tea made from the same plant as green and black tea. The way the tea is prepared differs: Black tea is permitted to oxidize until it turns black, whereas green tea is not. Oolong tea is partially oxidized because it falls somewhere in between the two. The color and distinctive flavor of oolong tea are the result of this partial oxidation.

Oolong tea is striking for containing l-theanine, an amino corrosive that diminishes nervousness and expands readiness and consideration. L-Polyphenols, which have been linked to lowering inflammation, preventing the growth of cancer, and lowering the risk of type 2 diabetes, are also abundant in oolong tea.

Teas to Avoid

 While the majority of teas are good for your health, you should avoid the following:
• Detox teas
designed for fad diets that promise quick weight loss. Laxatives that are potentially harmful to your health are frequently included in these teas.
• High-end tea lattes and beverages from your preferred department store chain. Even though some of these drinks, like the green tea latte, appear to be healthy, they are high in sugar.
• Trendy bubble teas that also have a lot of sugar, calories, and carbs and arent very healthy.
• Herbal teas that might make allergies worse. Numerous natural teas contain various sorts of organic products, spices, flavors and blossoms that certain individuals are hypersensitive to. Before consuming a new herbal tea, always read the packages ingredients if you have allergies.

10 Health Benefits of Drinking Lemon and Green
Tea

Green tea is a calming beverage that can be taken
anytime of day. Its flavorful, delicious, and simple
to make. Additionally, research has shown that it is
linked to a long list of potential health benefits, in
addition to being extremely nutritious.
The top ten health benefits of green tea with lemon
are listed below.

1. High in antioxidants both lemons and
    green tea contain a lot of antioxidants,
    which are substances that protect cells
    from oxidative damage and inflammation.

2.

Green tea, specifically, is wealthy in cell
reinforcements, for example, epigallocatechin
gallate (EGCG), quercetin, chlorogenic corrosive,
and theogallin. The antioxidants ascorbic acid,
hesperidin, naringin, and ferulic acid are all found in
abundance in lemons.

Research proposes cell reinforcements assume a
critical part in wellbeing and sickness and may
safeguard against constant circumstances, including
coronary illness, diabetes, disease, and heftiness.

Lemons and green tea both contain a lot of antioxidants, which can help prevent inflammation and other chronic conditions.

2. Advances weight reduction

Green tea with lemon can be an extraordinary expansion to a solid weight reduction diet. In fact, a number of studies have shown that green tea can help people lose weight and burn more fat.
One review of 15 studies found that drinking green tea with higher levels of EGCG for at least 12 weeks led to weight and fat loss.

In addition, 115 women in a study found that taking green tea extract for 12 weeks led to significant weight, BMI, and belly fat reductions. Despite the fact that researchers need to do more research in people, a few examinations propose that lemons could likewise advance weight reduction.

One study on animals found that treating mice with citrus flavonoids reduced the size of their fat cells. In mice fed a high fat diet, the citrus flavonoids also increased metabolism. Another study on animals found that feeding mice lemon polyphenols on a diet high in fat prevented them from gaining weight and storing fat. Studies recommend that drinking green tea might assist with diminishing body weight and muscle versus fat. Certain lemon compounds may also help prevent weight gain, according to some animal studies.

3. Improves blood sugar control and protects against type 2 diabetes, according to some research, which is interesting

Tea consumption has been linked to a lower risk of type 2 diabetes and complications related to diabetes, according to one review. Regular tea consumption may also improve insulin sensitivity and reduce inflammation in the body. The hormone that moves sugar into cells from the bloodstream is called insulin.

Green tea extract was found to reduce insulin resistance after 16 weeks of use in a study involving 92 people with type 2 diabetes. This might support better control of blood sugar. However, there is a need for additional research on the relationship between diabetes and green tea because other studies have yielded conflicting results.

4. May improve heart health Research has shown that lemons and green tea both have a number of health benefits for the heart

In point of fact, citrus flavonoids, such as those found in lemons, were mentioned in one review as having the potential to support healthy cholesterol levels, reduce inflammation, and improve the function of blood vessels.

Another study found that people who walked regularly and consumed lemons daily had lower blood pressure levels.
In a similar vein, a comparison of nine studies revealed that individuals who drank green tea on a regular basis had a lower risk of heart disease, stroke, and heart attack than those who did not.

In addition, a recent review of 24 studies revealed that drinking green tea may assist in lowering high systolic and diastolic blood pressure, which are both risk factors for heart disease. Consuming lemons and green tea together has been shown to reduce risk factors for heart disease and improve cardiovascular health.

5. Boosts brain health

Despite the need for more human research, some
studies suggest that lemon and green tea may offer a
number of potential advantages for brain health.
For example, a review of eight studies found that
drinking green tea reduced the risk of dementia and
cognitive impairment in some studies.

According to a different study, drinking green tea on
a regular basis may boost the metabolism of some
proteins that contribute to Alzheimers disease.
Citrus fruit compounds have also been found to
reduce inflammation, protect brain function, and
prevent plaque buildup in the brain, which could
contribute to Alzheimers disease, in animal and test
tube studies.

Green tea has been linked to a lower risk of
dementia, Alzheimers disease, and impaired brain
function. Lemon compounds may also help prevent
Alzheimers disease and improve brain function,
according to animal and test tube studies.

6. Lemons are a great source of vitamin C, a water-
soluble micronutrient with potent antioxidant
properties that may improve immunity

By improving immune cell function and reducing inflammation, vitamin C is essential to the immune system.

Vitamin C supplementation may also aid in the treatment and prevention of numerous respiratory and systemic infections.
In addition, certain compounds in green tea, such as EGCG, have been found to improve immune function and protect against autoimmune diseases like multiple sclerosis in animal studies.

Additionally, lemons and green tea contain a lot of antioxidants, which support a strong immune system. Vitamin C, which can help treat and prevent infections and reduce inflammation, is abundant in lemons. Green teas EGCG and other compounds may also help the immune system function better.

7. Boosts energy levels

Green tea is a natural source of caffeine, a stimulant for the central nervous system that many people take to get more energy.
Caffeine has been shown to boost mental and physical performance as well as combat fatigue, according to studies.

Caffeine has also been shown in some studies to increase endurance and athletic performance.

Green tea with lemon may be a good choice for people who are sensitive to the effects of high doses of caffeine because it contains less caffeine than coffee or energy drinks. Caffeine in green tea has been shown to reduce fatigue, increase alertness, and improve cognitive and physical functioning.

8. May aid in the prevention of kidney stones

Kidney stones are hard mineral deposits that can form in the kidneys and cause pain, nausea, and frequent urination.
A great way to help prevent kidney stones is to drink green tea with lemon. As a matter of fact, one enormous investigation discovered that drinking green tea was connected to a lower chance of creating kidney stones, particularly among men.

Lemons citric acid may also help prevent kidney stones by binding to calcium oxalate and increasing urine volume. This stops crystals from building up, which prevents kidney stones from forming.

One study found that taking just 4 ounces (118 milliliters) of lemon juice per day could help treat kidney stones.
There may be a link between drinking green tea and a lower risk of kidney stones. Citric acid in lemon juice may also aid in the prevention of kidney stones.

9. May help protect against cancer

Lemons and green tea may both have potent anti-cancer properties. A number of studies conducted in a test tube suggest that certain lemon-derived compounds may aid in stopping the growth and spread of cancer cells. Consuming more citrus fruits may also lower ones risk of several types of cancer, including breast, stomach, lung, and esophageal cancers, according to some studies.

Green tea has also been found to lower cancer risk in research. Specifically, studies recommend that green tea might help safeguard against bladder, bosom, colorectal, and prostate disease cells.
Lemons and green tea, according to some studies, may slow the growth and spread of various types of cancer cells.

10. Keeps you hydrated

Drinking lemon-infused green tea can help you stay hydrated. Nearly every aspect of health depends on getting enough water. Its especially important for skin health, losing weight, brain health, digestive health, and kidney health. Even kidney stones, headaches, and constipation can be avoided by drinking enough fluids every day. Lemon and green tea can help you stay hydrated, which could support a variety of health issues.

Green tea with lemon is not difficult to make at home by blending green tea and adding newly crushed lemon juice.
Green tea with lemon might accompany a few medical advantages. It might help you lose weight, keep you hydrated, give you more energy, and help your brain, heart, and immune system stay healthy. Spices and herbs have long been used to enhance foods flavor, aroma, and appeal.

Chapter 9

Antioxidants found in vegetables, herbs, and spices that improve kidney function

There is now evidence to suggest that in addition to pleasing our palates, these pantry staples may also improve our health. Research shows likely advantages of flavors and spices, which are plentiful in cancer prevention agents and astounding wellsprings of different nutrients and minerals.

 More than 2,000 of the compounds found in herbs and spices have been identified by modern science, which has begun to investigate them. Some spices and herbs even have levels of nutrients comparable to those found in fruits and vegetables.

When you have flavorful alternatives that are also friendly to the kidneys, it is easier to reduce your intake of sugar, salt, and fat. You wont feel like youre missing anything this way. You dont have to wait for a special occasion to start changing up your diet because these spices and herbs are simple to incorporate into everyday meals.

Spice up your diet with these seven kidney-friendly seasonings:

Rosemary

This herb helps with memory, thinking, and brain health. Not certain how to utilize rosemary? Its simple. Olive oil should be applied to the tops of the frozen dinner rolls before baking, and crushed rosemary leaves should be sprinkled on top. You can also try adding a little oregano, thyme, and rosemary to chicken or vegetable soup to give it a Tuscan flavor.

Garlic

Garlic has antioxidant and antibacterial properties. Add garlic powder or crushed garlic to cooked pasta, rice, or vegetables for extra flavor and nutrients. Olive oil mixed with fresh garlic or garlic powder and brushed over Italian bread can also give garlic bread a healthy makeover. The bread should be grilled for two to three minutes.

Oregano

Like many leafy greens, contains a lot of vitamin K, which is good for your bones and blood.For that classic "pizza flavor" without the potassium of tomatoes, sprinkle oregano on your garlic bread. You can also easily add herbs to stir fries and pasta by combining oregano and garlic powder.

Chili

Chili peppers contain a lot of vitamin A, which is good for the skin and eyes. Ongoing exploration has shown that consuming chilies may likewise give your digestion a lift. There are numerous ways to include chilies in your diet without burning your tongue if you typically avoid spicy foods.

There is a "spice spectrum" to help you distinguish mild chilies from spicy ones. In order of severity: Some chilies to try are cayenne, crushed red pepper, black pepper, and paprika. Sprinkling paprika on deviled eggs, tuna or chicken salad, or adding cayenne pepper to your favorite vinaigrette are easy ways to include them in your diet. Please be aware

that people with kidney failure should avoid taking
more vitamin A.

Ginger

This root has been shown to ease nausea and aid
digestion. Ginger is an excellent addition to your
diet because of its numerous anti-inflammatory,
antioxidant, and pain-relieving properties. Ginger
can be easily added to marinades for fish and
poultry, as it is in many Asian dishes. It could
actually be added to organic product plates of mixed
greens and it supplements green tea and lemonade.

Cinnamon

This spice may help regulate blood sugar, according
to recent research. For a delicious and nutritious
snack, cinnamon can be easily added to applesauce,
cream of wheat, or even sliced raw or baked apples.

Basil: Basil imparts flavor without significantly
increasing potassium or phosphorus levels. Basil can
easily be included in everyday meals. On a
sandwich, substitute basil leaves for lettuce, or shred
them and use them as a garnish.

Spices And Flavors

Spices and flavors are a decent option in contrast to the pre-made flavors that are accessible in your nearby store. Most pre-made seasonings have a lot of sodium, which is bad for people who have kidney disease. As a result, patients can choose to make their own mixes of spices and herbs for much less money and for better health.

It is essential to comprehend the distinctions between seeds, spices, and herbs.

Herbs

The fragrant flowers and leaves of plants are the
source of herbs. Some herbs, like savory, thyme,
sweet basil, marjoram, and oregano, come from the
mint family, while others, like rosemary and bay
leaf, come from a type of evergreen.

Spices

Flavors are gotten from the stem, root, seeds, bark
or bulbs of the plant. Instances of flavors are
cinnamon, cloves and ginger.

Seeds

These can be seeds or small, whole fruits. Caraway,
dill, cumin, and fennel are the fruits that belong to
the parsley family. Mustard is the seed of a plant in
the cabbage family. Options that are good for the
kidneys include the following spices, herbs, and
seeds that are safe for patients:

Allspice, bay leaf, caraway, cardamom, cayenne,
chili, curry, dill, ginger, marjoram, mint, mustard,
oregano, paprika, parsley, rosemary, savory, tartar,

and thyme. Dillweed, chili powder, onion powder, garlic powder, and chili flakes should be avoided in blends, herbs, and spices.
Salt, sugar, ethoxyquin, maltodextrin, citric acid, hydrogenated cottonseed oil, silicon dioxide, and spice extract are all ingredients in the flavoring.

Chapter 10

How olive leaf extract and omega-3 fatty acids can improve kidney function.

Uremic pruritus, more accurately referred to as "chronic kidney disease-associated pruritus" (CKD-aP), continues to be one of the most debilitating, frequent, and potentially disabling conditions in patients with advanced or end-stage renal disease (ESRD).

It affects 15%-49% of pre-dialysis CKD patients and 50%-90% of those on dialysis, including peritoneal dialysis and hemodialysis (HD). In some patients, the degree of itching varies and appears to be cyclical; However, it does not resolve everything. During the day and at night, itching can range from sporadic disturbance to complete agitation.

In most cases, CKD-aP is more severe at night than during the day. The skin of 25% of affected patients initially appears dry and scaly, similar to that of subjects without pruritus, likely as a result of hypersensitivity reactions against dialysis membranes.

During or immediately following dialysis. In contrast to dermatological itch, uremic pruritus has a significant impact on quality of life because it causes severe discomfort, anxiety, depression, and sleep disorders.

However, linear crusts, excoriations with or without impetigo, papules, ulcerations, and, less frequently, prurigo nodularis may be observed as secondary skin lesions due to severe scratching.

Generalized pruritus is the predominant complaint in 25 to 50 percent of patients, whereas CKD Chronic fatigue, disruptions in the day-night rhythm, and impairments in mental and physical capacity are all associated with poor quality sleep.

Unfortunately, there are few treatment options for CKD-aP. Legitimacy of most examinations regarding this matter remaining parts sketchy as a result of unfortunate documentation of the essentials, of corresponding infections and treatments taken, and of tiny review populace numbers. CKD-aP, on the other hand, frequently resists conventional treatments.

Indeed, numerous treatment options for pruritus have been investigated. Regular, intensive, and effective dialysis, the use of a non-complement-activating dialysis membrane, adherence to dietary restrictions, acupuncture, and ultraviolet B therapy are non-pharmacologic treatments for CKD-aP.

Capsaicin cream, endocannabinoid cream, tacrolimus ointment, antihistamines, gabapentin, naltrexone, nalfurafine, thalidomide, pentoxiphylline, activated charcoal, cholestyramine, epoetin, pizotyline, ketotifen, and nicergoline are among the pharmacological treatments that have been.

However, the essential fatty acids and their metabolites derived from the cyclooxygenase and lipoxygenase pathways, which include prostaglandins and leukotrienes, are of significant etiological interest in relation to CKD-aP.

ESRD patients are known to have abnormal fatty acid profiles and exhibit symptoms consistent with those associated with essential fatty acid deficiency, such as pruritus, abnormal perspiration, delayed wound healing Fish oil, which is high in omega-3 fatty acids, has been shown to be beneficial in the alleviation of pruritus.

These prospects suggest that dietary long chain omega-3 fatty acids may offer a therapeutic supplement for cutaneous inflammatory or itching disorders in CKD patients. Omega-3 fatty acids exert anti-inflammatory effects for many inflammatory disorders. In order to better understand the potential clinical benefits of omega-3 PUFA in the treatment of CKD-aP.

Conclusion

The kidneys serve as incredibly effective filters, removing waste and poisonous substances from the body while reintroducing vitamins, amino acids, glucose, hormones, and other essential nutrients into the bloodstream. High blood flow to the kidneys is filtered by highly specialized blood arteries.

Ones kidneys may fail suddenly or gradually although acute renal failure is frequently transient, it must be managed until kidney function is restored. Long-term development of chronic kidney disease is linked to a variety of risk factors, such as diabetes and high blood pressure. Early detection of chronic kidney disease can lengthen the lifespan of your kidneys with the help of medicines and lifestyle modifications. Dialysis, kidney transplantation, or non-dialysis comprehensive conservative care are all available treatments for kidney failure.

A considerable portion of individuals with chronic kidney disease never have a particular cause identified, and the illness progresses slowly. It has several multi-system consequences that greatly reduce sufferers quality of life and lengthen their mortality. Thus, it is crucial to avoid chronic kidney disease and identify it early.

For patients who are at a high risk of developing chronic renal disease, annual screening is advised. This include measuring the renal clearance function, examining blood pressure, and testing urine using a dipstick. Kidney preventive treatments are recommended for patients with chronic renal disease in order to stop or decrease the loss of kidney function.